Suicide and Self-harm

A Parent's Guide

Pamela Rose Rasmussen

Suicide and Self-harm
Copyright © 2023 by Pamela Rose Rasmussen

All rights reserved. No part of this publication may be reproduced, distributed, or transmitted in any form or by any means, including photocopying, recording, or other electronic or mechanical methods, without the prior written permission of the author, except in the case of brief quotations embodied in critical reviews and certain other non-commercial uses permitted by copyright law.

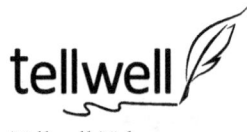

Tellwell Talent
www.tellwell.ca

ISBN
978-0-2288-9699-9 (Paperback)

Support Services

Hello Reader,

Throughout this book, we talk about suicidal ideation and self-harm. This information is directed at you, the parents and caregivers, so that you can best help the child or teen you are caring for. We cover topics of sexual assault, domestic/family violence, physical assault, mental health, and suicidal ideation/self-harming. I understand that some readers may find some or all of these topics confronting for many reasons. Below is a list of numbers and websites you can call or reach out to online for support. Remember you are never alone; there is always help for you and your child. There is always someone who cares, who wants to listen, and who can help.

Family/Domestic Violence and Sexual Assault Counselling

1800 555 677
www.1800respect.org.au

Lifeline Counselling Services
13 11 14
www.lifeline.org.au

Mental Health Line
1800 011 511

Kids Helpline (from five to twenty-five years old)
1800 55 1800

In an emergency, call police, fire, or ambulance
000
For non-urgent help, call police at
131 444

Table of Contents

Chapter one 1

Chapter two 11

Chapter three 27

References 43

Chapter one

Suicidal ideation in children and teenagers

What is the cause?

Regrettably, suicide among children and teenagers constitutes a grave issue. It stands as the second-most common cause of death for individuals aged ten to fourteen years old.

Several factors can lead to suicidal thoughts in children and teenagers. These encompass but are not limited to:

Depression	Sadness
Confusion	Anger
Attention	Anxiety
Stress	Self-doubt
Pressure to succeed	Financial uncertainty
Disappointment	Loss/grief

Further along in the text, we explore these factors on an individual basis.

Most children and teenagers who attempt suicide are grappling with a significant mental health disorder, typically depression. In the case of younger children and preteens, suicide attempts are often impulsive.

It is crucial to treat any suicidal thoughts, feelings, or actions exhibited by children and teenagers with utmost seriousness. Prompt recognition and diagnosis of their illness is necessary, followed by suitable treatment for their age group administered by qualified professionals.

While suicide ideation is frequently linked to depression, other risk factors may contribute as well. These could include but are not limited to:

Sexual abuse/assault	Physical abuse/assault
Family history of suicide attempts	Exposure to any sort of violence
Impulsivity	Aggressive or disruptive behaviour
Access to firearms	Bullying from others
Feelings of hopelessness or helplessness	Acute loss or rejection

In some instances, children and teens might openly express their suicidal thoughts. Other times, they might not. Those who do might utter statements such as, "I wish I were dead" or "I won't be a problem for you much longer." However, it's much more challenging to discern such ideations in those who don't verbalize their feelings. Parents can be vigilant for certain warning signs that could indicate a child or teen is harbouring suicidal thoughts. These include but are not limited to:

Changes in eating or sleeping habits	Frequent or pervasive sadness
Withdrawal from friends, family, and regular activities	Frequent complaints about physical symptoms often related to emotions, such as stomachaches, headaches, fatigue, etc.
Decline in the quality of schoolwork	Preoccupation with death and dying

In certain cases, if a child or teen is contemplating suicide and has intentions to act on it, they may discontinue talking and planning for their future, behaving externally as if the thought doesn't exist. They may also begin to give away their significant possessions.

Discussing suicide with your child or teen can be an exceptionally challenging task. Some parents might prefer to avoid this conversation, delegating it to someone else instead. If you're concerned for your child's safety, consulting health professionals is a prudent course of action. However, initiating this conversation yourself could potentially facilitate your child's willingness to confide in you, as a parent. If you observe any warning signs, you could broach the subject accordingly. For instance, you could say, "I've noticed that you no longer seem to be planning for your future. Are you contemplating harming or even ending your life?" or "Lately, you seem to be struggling and have become more distant than usual. I'm here to listen. Are you feeling sad or depressed?" This dialogue ensures your child or teen recognizes that they can trust you and that you're a safe haven for them. After establishing this connection, you can seek appropriate professional help.

Please note that raising such questions doesn't implant ideas into your child's mind; instead, it fosters a safe and caring environment, which is precisely what they need at this time. They may have already been exposed to such concepts through conversations with friends at school, but it's crucial for them to feel they can trust their parents and be open about their experiences.

If it's suspected that a child or teen is suicidal, parents, teachers, coaches and other adults in their life like family members, etc. should always prioritize caution and safety. Immediate evaluation by a trained and qualified mental health professional is of utmost importance.

Furthermore, parents must strive to remain calm when dealing with a suicidal child. Anger or strong emotional reactions could potentially exacerbate the situation and won't be beneficial for any of the parties involved. If you as the parent or caregiver feel that you cannot adequately handle the conversation with the child or teen who is suicidal, then it is in the child's or teen's best interest to seek help from someone you trust who can approach the conversation in a more delicate way.

What is self-harming?

Self-harm, also referred to as self-injury, self-mutilation, or self-abuse, occurs when individuals intentionally inflict pain upon themselves without the aim of suicide. Health professionals frequently label actions such as cutting and other forms of self-harm as non-suicidal self-injury.

It's crucial to understand that if a child or teen begins to self-harm, it doesn't necessarily indicate they are contemplating suicide or that they have a desire to die. However, recent research suggests that if non-suicidal self-injury persists over an extended period, it can elevate the risk of suicidal thoughts and behaviours in children and teens. Therefore, parents and caregivers must promptly intervene if they suspect that their child or teen is self-harming.

While children and teens who self-harm may not be considering suicide, such actions could unintentionally result in self-inflicted death if taken too far. Therefore, it's important not to pass judgement on a child or teen who engages in self-harm but to provide support and assistance instead.

How do parents react?

When confronted with indications that their child or teen is engaging in self-harm, parents and caregivers may feel a mix of confusion, anger, guilt, self-doubt, shame, and helplessness. While they understand the immediate need for assistance, they might be unsure of where to start. It's vital that parents resist the urge to react with anger towards a child or teen who is self-harming; there's always an underlying cause for such behaviour. As with suicidal children and teens, those who self-harm require a safe environment and trustworthy individuals to confide in about their experiences. This book provides various methods that parents and caregivers can utilize to support children and teens during their struggles.

Parents may not know which signs to watch out for when it comes to self-harming behaviours. Here are a few indications to be mindful of if you're concerned about your child:

- The most prevalent form of non-suicidal self-injury is skin cutting, so you may notice cuts or scars on your child's hands, wrists, stomach, legs, or other body parts. These may be deep wounds or numerous smaller cuts in a single area. However, it's crucial to note that children often conceal their injuries by wearing extensive jewellery or long sleeves even in warm weather, and so these cuts and scars might not be immediately noticeable.

- Other methods of self-injury can involve head-banging, burning, hair-pulling, or excessively scratching the skin until it bleeds. Some children might punch themselves, insert objects into their bodies, consume harmful substances like bleach or detergent, or deliberately try to break their own bones. In some instances, children or teens may self-harm only once, but those who persistently engage in non-suicidal self-injury often employ multiple methods.

What causes self-harm in children/teens?

In some instances, there's no singular identifiable cause for self-harm. However, children and teens who engage in self-harm frequently experience intense emotional distress. Some report feelings of loneliness, worthlessness, or emptiness and they resort to any means to alleviate these feelings, even momentarily. Others express feeling overstimulated, misunderstood, or anxious about forming close relationships. Some feel burdened by school and family responsibilities. Some harbour a desire to punish themselves for self-perceived wrongdoings. If a child or teen is experiencing physical or sexual violence, they may feel unable to disclose it to anyone and might resort to self-harm as their only outlet, keeping the violence and self-harming a secret. Self-harm can also represent a method for children to exert control over their bodies when they perceive a lack of control in other areas or when other aspects of their lives feel unmanageable.

Female children and teens who self-harm tend to gravitate towards cutting, while their male counterparts are more likely to inflict harm by hitting themselves. However, self-harm is not gender-exclusive; children of all gender identities, including males and those who identify as nonbinary or transgender, engage in non-suicidal self-harm.

Self-harm vs suicide

Most instances of self-harm arise from a temporary desire to escape rather than a longing for death. However, teens who struggle to cease non-suicidal self-harm encounter significantly higher rates of suicidal ideation and are more likely to die by suicide compared to their peers who do not self-harm. Self-harm tends to peak during the teen years, with many teens discontinuing the behaviour as they navigate beyond this period.

How can I help my child?

The approach for addressing self-harm in children and teens mirrors that of handling suicidal thoughts. It's crucial to initiate a conversation with them, no matter how challenging it might be for you, as it's undoubtedly more difficult for them. Don't hesitate to enquire if they are involved in non-suicidal self-harm or if they know anyone who is. Adopt a non-judgemental stance, emphasizing active listening over speaking. It's acceptable to acknowledge the discomfort of the topic, but make sure to express your care and concern: "This is difficult for me to contemplate as I care deeply for you and desire your safety and health at all times."

Be prepared for strong reactions from the child or teen. As individuals engaging in non-suicidal self-harm often deny and attempt to conceal this behaviour, your child might become upset or refuse to discuss it. In a calmer moment, express your concerns about their potential self-harming behaviour and your intention to consult a doctor. Encourage their presence during this discussion, but proceed with the appointment even if they resist. You can try and explain to the child or teen how important it is to seek professional help as they would have a better understanding about suicide/self-harm than you as the parent or caregiver. Alternatively, you can get another trusted adult to have a conversation with the child or teen in their home environment and see if they might feel more comfortable going with them to seek professional help. The most important thing is to let your child or teen know that under no circumstances have they done anything wrong and that you are simply acting for their best interest.

It's important to trust your healthcare provider. Paediatricians, who focus on children's health, are typically knowledgeable about non-suicidal self-harm due to their experience treating similar cases. Neither shame nor blame should be associated with your child's struggles. Allow private time for your child to converse with their doctor. The doctor can work alongside you and your child to develop a tailored care plan, possibly involving talk or play therapy, stress-reduction methods, medication, or other effective strategies.

Creating a safer home environment can also support your child. If your child is self-harming, removing potential hazards such as sharp objects, poisons, or weapons can help. While it may be challenging to eliminate all risk all the time, it's particularly vital during periods of expressed self-harm urges or high stress. Keep firearms inaccessible and medications locked away, especially if your child expresses suicidal thoughts. Discuss a safety plan with your healthcare provider, encompassing practical measures for securing your home and handling emergencies.

Prioritize your family's wellbeing. If your family is consistently facing high stress levels, consider ways to alleviate this. It's important for children and teens to feel they can request downtime without guilt, understanding that self-care take precedence over academic or extracurricular obligations. Some children and their families are more susceptible to mental health issues due to factors such as trauma, violence, unstable family dynamics, and poverty. A supportive parent-child relationship can provide significant safety and foster resilience in children facing adversity.

Maintain transparency with your child. Your child's welfare depends on a network of support from family, teachers, coaches, and others, so it's essential to not keep their struggles hidden. Share relevant information while respecting your child's privacy, and seek guidance from your doctor on appropriate disclosure methods. Educate others about your child's situation to ensure cohesive support. It might be a good idea to inform your child of this information being shared so they know who they can trust if they don't feel safe within themselves at any point in time. If your child or teen becomes angry because of the information shared, it is important that you as the parent or caregiver sit down and have a conversation with them about why you felt the need to share this information. Then, find out why the child or teen feels the way they do. Open communication here is the key.

Remember, self-harm doesn't equate to a desire for death, nor does it make you a bad parent. Similar to any health issue, your hopeful outlook, commitment to treatment, and unconditional love can significantly assist your child's recovery.

Chapter two

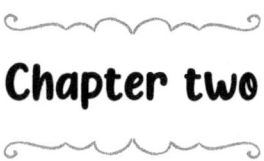

Definitions and effects

What is depression?

Depression is a prevalent and severe health condition that adversely influences your emotions, thoughts, and actions. However, it's important to remember that depression is treatable. Symptoms of depression can include persistent feelings of sadness or a diminished interest in previously enjoyed activities. This condition can result in various emotional and physical issues, reducing one's capacity to perform effectively at work, school, or home.

To be diagnosed with depression, the symptoms must persist for at least two weeks and must denote a change from your usual state of functioning. While both children and teens can experience depression, their display of symptoms can differ from adults. Their symptoms may centre around sadness, a sense of despair, mood changes, irritability, or sudden episodes of anger, which may seem like a low mood or sadness in adults.

The severity of other depression symptoms can range from mild to severe and can encompass:

- Experiencing a constant feeling of sadness or depressed mood

- Losing interest in or deriving less pleasure from activities once enjoyed

- Experiencing changes in appetite, leading to either weight loss or gain unrelated to diet

- Having sleep disturbances or excessive sleep

- Feeling drained or noticeably more fatigued

- Exhibiting an increase in aimless physical activities (like restlessness, pacing, slowed movements or speech that are noticeable to others, or changes in handwriting) (Mental health problems like depression can cause handwriting changes. For instance, a girl's handwriting worsened noticeably when she became severely depressed.)

- Withdrawing from social interactions with family and friends

- Experiencing feelings of worthlessness or guilt

- Struggling with thinking, concentrating, or making decisions

- Having thoughts about death or suicide

Several risk factors could contribute to the onset of depression, including:

- Trauma experienced during childhood or teen years

- Biochemistry, as variances in certain brain chemicals could result in depressive symptoms

- Genetics, as depression tends to be familial; for instance, if one identical twin is diagnosed with depression, the other twin has a 70% likelihood of experiencing the disorder at some point in their life

- Personality, as individuals with low self-esteem, who are more susceptible to stress, or who generally have a pessimistic outlook are more likely to experience depression

- Environmental factors, as persistent exposure to violence, neglect, abuse, or poverty can increase the vulnerability to depression for some individuals

How is childhood depression treated?

The treatment approach for depression in children and teens is quite similar to that for adults. It typically involves psychotherapy, commonly known as counselling. Depending on the child's age, the therapy could be talk therapy or play therapy. The latter is often more effective with younger children as they find it easier to express their thoughts and feelings through play.

Medication may also be part of the treatment plan. A healthcare provider might recommend starting with psychotherapy, and then considering antidepressant medication if the symptoms are severe or if there's no significant improvement with counselling alone. Many medical professionals assert that combining psychotherapy with medication yields the most effective results in managing childhood depression.

However, like any other treatment, antidepressants come with a caution; they might increase the risk of suicidal ideation and behaviour in children and teens suffering from depression and other mental health disorders. If you have any queries or concerns regarding this, it's advisable to have a discussion with your child's doctor to be provided with the necessary clarification and guidance.

What is the difference between depression and sadness?

Sadness is an inherent human emotion that everyone experiences at certain moments in life. It is a natural response to circumstances that bring about emotional distress or hurt. The intensity of sadness can vary, but like other emotions, it is typically fleeting and diminishes with time, making it different from depression.

Depression, on the other hand, is a persistent mental health condition. It interferes with social, occupational, and other significant aspects of daily life. If not treated, the symptoms of depression can linger for a prolonged period. Depression may include feeling:

- Overwhelmed or indecisive

- Guilty
- Irritable or frustrated
- Lack of confidence
- Unhappy or disappointed
- Miserable or sad

During periods of sadness, the feeling might seem all-consuming. However, during times of sadness, there are usually instances when one is able to experience joy or find comfort. This contrasts with depression, where the feelings one endures permeate all areas of life. It can become difficult or even impossible to find pleasure in anything, including previously enjoyed activities and individuals. Depression is a mental health disorder, not just an emotion.

Confusion in children/teens

Much like adults, children and teens can also experience confusion. They might struggle with their sense of location, time, the people around them, or even their own identity. Other signs that align with this state of confusion are agitation, restlessness, hallucinatory behaviour such as picking at non-existent items, emotional distress that doesn't respond to usual comfort strategies, and problems with attention or memory.

Parents can identify signs of confusion in their children. These signs include difficulties with short-term memory, problems completing tasks, diminished attention span, incoherent speech, and trouble keeping up with conversations. Sometimes, this state of confusion can be temporary and will resolve over time. However, in other instances, confusion can persist and be indicative of a chronic condition.

Anger in children/teens

Children and teens demonstrating escalating aggression, hostility, or violence towards others might be grappling with a mood disorder, such as depression, or a behavioural issue, such as conduct disorder. Children and teens who find it hard to control their anger and frustration could benefit from learning anger management skills. These skills can be imparted via individual and family therapy sessions. These strategies might be all that's necessary to assist the child or teen in managing their impulsive behaviour, and challenging their frustration in a more socially acceptable way.

The part of the brain called the limbic region, responsible for executive functions, can be underdeveloped in children and teens. This affects their judgement, emotional regulation, decision-making, and self-control. As their brains are still developing, children might express their anger when they feel slighted, let down, or frustrated, as they lack the yet-to-be-developed coping skills.

Children and teens may harbour internalized feelings of despair and worthlessness, unknown to others, that could stem from past traumatic experiences like abuse. These feelings can engender shame, severe self-criticism, and self-punishment – all commonly associated with depression.

The connection between anger and depression in children and teens can be complex since they may not always communicate their troubles to an adult. So, how does a parent discern that their child or teen's mood swings have escalated to a severe mental health risk?

In the midst of a psychiatric crisis, the child or teen might show the following indicators of emotional distress:

- Exhibiting aggressive or violent behaviour
- Losing interest in social and extracurricular activities
- Running away from home or skipping school
- Showing extreme sadness or despair
- Engaging in illegal or risky activities
- Frequently skipping school
- Displaying extreme irritability or agitation
- Experiencing disruptions in sleep
- Becoming more secretive or isolated
- Experiencing a sudden decline in academic performance
- Engaging in self-harm
- Abusing substances
- Expressing suicidal thoughts or making suicide threats

Attention in children/teens

Patients diagnosed with major depressive disorder frequently report struggles with focus and concentration that adversely affect their daily routines. Current primary treatments often don't effectively mitigate these issues.

If medications and psychotherapy, which are traditional treatment methods for mental health conditions, are not yielding positive results or improving your child's or teen's condition, it might be time to discuss alternative or additional treatment options with a psychiatrist. These additional options could include:

1. Adjustment of Current Medications★★: Your psychiatrist may suggest adjusting the dosage or the type of medication your child or teen is taking. There are numerous drugs available, and sometimes it takes trial and error to find the right one.

2. Incorporation of New Therapies★★: There are many types of therapy aside from traditional talk therapy. Cognitive-behavioural therapy, dialectical behaviour therapy, and family therapy are just a few examples. You might also consider group therapy for your child or teen, which can provide support from peers experiencing similar challenges.

3. Electroconvulsive Therapy (ECT)★★: Although it's not a first-line treatment, ECT can be very effective for individuals who do not respond to medications or psychotherapy, particularly those with severe depression or suicidal thoughts.

4. **Lifestyle Modifications**★★: Sometimes, changes in diet, exercise, sleep habits, and reducing alcohol or caffeine can enhance the effectiveness of mental health treatments. Mindfulness and relaxation techniques can also be beneficial.

Remember, it's crucial to maintain an open dialogue with your psychiatrist about your child's or teen's treatment. Discuss any side effects from medications, feelings towards therapy, or any changes in your child's or teen's condition. This information can help your child's or teen's psychiatrist create the most effective treatment plan for your child or teen.

Why is attention so pivotal in mental health?

Regardless of whether it's depression or any other mental health disorder, attention plays a crucial role. Attention is fundamental in nearly every aspect of life, including education, work, and personal relationships. Attention facilitates the concentration required to process information and form memories. Moreover, attention helps individuals ignore distractions, enabling them to concentrate on and accomplish specific tasks.

Anxiety in children/teens

It's not uncommon for children to experience fears, concerns, and occasional feelings of sadness or despair. Intense fears may rise at different stages of their development. For instance, toddlers often experience significant distress when separated from their parents, even when they are safe and well-cared for. While these fears and concerns are normal in children, if they persist or become extreme, they could indicate anxiety or depression.

If a child doesn't grow out of the fears typical of young children, or if their worries are so numerous that they interfere with school, homelife, or play, they may be diagnosed with an anxiety disorder. Various types of anxiety disorders can manifest in different ways, such as:

- Intense fear when separated from parents (separation anxiety)
- Extreme fear of specific objects or situations, such as dogs, insects, or doctor visits (phobias)
- Significant fear of school and other social environments (social anxiety)
- Persistent worry about the future or potential negative events (general anxiety)
- Experiencing reoccurring episodes of sudden, unexpected, intense fear accompanied by symptoms like racing heart, breathing difficulties, dizziness, shakiness, or sweating (panic disorder)

Certain social factors can further exacerbate anxiety in children and teens. These include experiences of peer exclusion, bullying, witnessing domestic violence, parents' substance misuse, bereavement, and family disruption.

Anxiety might manifest as fear or worry but can also lead to irritability and anger in children. Symptoms of anxiety can also include difficulty sleeping, as well as physical symptoms such as fatigue, headaches, or stomachaches. Some children may internalize their worries, making it easy to overlook their symptoms. If you suspect your child or teen might be dealing with anxiety, it's important to have an open conversation with them about it and seek advice from your healthcare provider.

Stress in children/teens

Stress in childhood can occur in any situation that necessitates the child to adjust or change. While positive changes, like starting a new venture, can trigger stress, stress is often associated more with negative life alterations such as family member's illness or death.

For teens, sources of stress can range from social issues like disputes with friends, bullying, or peer pressure to personal challenges such as becoming sexually active or feeling pressured to do so. Other factors like changing schools, relocating, or dealing with housing instability or homelessness can also cause stress. Negative self-perception can further contribute to a teen's stress levels.

Prolonged or toxic stress can have severe consequences for a child's health, increasing their risk of obesity, diabetes, heart disease, and certain cancers among other conditions. Additionally, it heightens their susceptibility to mental health issues like depression, as well as substance abuse, smoking, teenage pregnancy, sexually-transmitted infections, suicidal tendencies, and domestic violence.

Thus, it's crucial to help children and teens manage their stress effectively. Here are some strategies that might assist in reducing stress levels:

- Prioritize good sleep: Adequate sleep is critical for maintaining physical and emotional health.

- Encourage physical activity: Exercise is a powerful stress reducer for people of all age groups.

- Facilitate open conversations: Discussing stressors with your child or teen could lead to problem-solving strategies they might not have considered.

- Foster a relaxing environment: Children and teens tend to feel more relaxed in environments that promote fun and tranquillity.

- Spend time outdoors: Engaging in family activities like picnics or outdoor games can help reduce stress.

- Promote journalling: Encourage your child or teen to write about their concerns as a way of processing their feelings.

- Teach mindfulness: Mindfulness practices are effective stress reducers and beneficial for all age groups.

Self-doubt in children/teens

Negative emotions are intricately connected with self-doubt. Indeed, children and teens who have experienced high levels of anxiety and depression are more susceptible to feelings of self-doubt. Past experiences that were distressing can contribute to self-doubt long after the individual believes the issue has been resolved.

Self-doubt and low self-esteem often occur together, and some signs that a child or teen might be grappling with these issues include:

- Speaking negatively about themselves or expressing self-criticism
- Self-deprecating humour
- Overemphasis on their shortcomings while overlooking their accomplishments
- Tendency to blame themselves for mishaps, even when it's beyond their control
- Believing that others are superior to them
- Feeling undeserving of enjoyment or pleasure

Certain triggers can lead a child or teen to develop self-doubt. These might include:

- An unhappy childhood marked by extremely critical parents, teachers, or other significant figures
- Poor academic performance, leading to diminished confidence
- Prolonged stressful life events such as a relationship breakdown or financial difficulties (particularly relevant for working teens)

Pressure to succeed felt by children/teens

The majority of pressure felt by children and teens often emanates from their parents or caregivers. Constant pressure from these figures can induce defensive attitudes in children, potentially leading to the development of unhealthy habits, injuries, and mental illness that could persist into adulthood. As a parent or caregiver, it's crucial to recognize a child's abilities and provide guidance on how they can hone their talents.

Parental pressure can be categorized into two main forms: direct and indirect. Direct pressure can manifest as shouting, force, or constant complaints. On the other hand, indirect pressure might involve making your child feel guilty or reminding them of stringent expectations.

Parents rarely intend to exert undue pressure on their children or teens to achieve success, but it can inadvertently occur. As a parent, you could express your concerns about being unable to meet your child's/teen's expectations. Share your future vision of what you see for yourself in say five years' time, even if it's still uncertain. Demonstrating that you are considering what lies ahead – even without clear direction – might help them feel more secure. It's essential to listen to their thoughts and feelings; every child needs to feel safe and listened to.

Financial uncertainty felt by children/teens

Children can become anxious about their family's financial situation if they overhear their parents discussing or arguing about money. This anxiety can be amplified if they are unable to afford the same commodities as their peers, such as clothing, food, or school supplies, or if they are unable to socialize to the same degree. Such financial worries can make children feel guilty and helpless, impacting their confidence and self-worth.

Parents' financial instability can negatively affect children's and teens' development. When parents continually struggle to manage family finances, navigate bureaucratic systems, or make difficult decisions about expenditure on their children, they may experience heightened stress. This added strain can result in decreased energy for consistent interaction with and supervision of their children.

Disappointment felt by children/teens

Children can experience disappointment due to a myriad of reasons on any given day. They might feel let down if they can't have their preferred snack or if they miss out on spending time with a friend. Unfulfilled expectations during birthday parties or holiday celebrations can also trigger disappointment.

People often feel disappointed when their expectations or perceptions don't align with reality. They might have set their expectations or hopes for others too high, considering the circumstances. Even though they might believe that their expectations are fair and achievable, they may not always be realistic.

Loss for children/teens

Loss can mean different things to different people. Some examples of loss are:

- Physical loss like the death of someone they know or were close with by natural causes or by suicide or murder

- Social loss like their parents' divorce or end of relationship or loss of an important friendship, ill health, loss of a job, or being isolated by one's own family

When it comes to loss and grief, there is no right or wrong way for any one person to act. Everyone deals with situations differently and processes them differently and at different times and stages.

Some of the emotional reactions of children, teens, and even adults are:

- Anger
- Guilt
- Anxiety
- Sadness
- Despair
- Suicidal ideation
- Self-harming behaviour
- Withdrawal from others and things they normally like to do
- Difficulty concentrating at school

Chapter three

Other risk factors

Other risk factors can contribute to suicidal ideation and self-harming behaviour. Here we look into what they are and how they impact children and teens.

What is sexual abuse/assault?

Sexual abuse is defined as any form of sexual contact or behaviour occurring without consent.

- Sexual abuse may take the form of inappropriate touching, exposure to sexual acts or pornographic materials, or using the Internet for grooming. Perpetrators of this abuse upon a child or an adult can include family members, partners, neighbours, sports coaches, teachers, strangers, and any member of the community.

Sexual assault can also include rape, which is sexual penetration of the mouth, anus, or vagina without consent.

- Sexual assault is related to sexual abuse. Sexual assault can also include threatening behaviour; violence; or forced, coercive, or exploitative behaviour. Reasons one may not be able to give consent include age, being unconscious or asleep, severe intoxication, having a developmental disability, or having mental health issues that significantly impair decision-making.

How can this affect children/teens?

Sexual abuse has been identified as a cause of post-traumatic stress disorder (PTSD) in children and teens, affecting them in five main areas:

- Health issues
- Psychological troubles
- Sexual problems
- Recurrent self-harm
- Chronic suicidal thoughts

Furthermore, sexual abuse can lead to the development of a variety of other issues in victims. These issues can include depression, anxiety, sleep disturbance, difficulty with physical contact, relationship problems, educational challenges, substance abuse, psychotic symptoms, antisocial behaviour, eating disorders, conduct disorders, and struggles with securing and maintaining employment.

What is physical abuse/assault?

Physical abuse/assault can involve:

- Scratching or biting

- Pushing or shoving
- Slapping
- Kicking
- Choking or strangling
- Throwing things
- Force-feeding or denying food
- Using weapons or objects to inflict hurt
- Physical restraint (such as pinning against a wall, floor, or bed)
- Reckless driving
- Other acts that threaten or cause hurt

How can this affect children/teens?

The immediate or primary effects of physical abuse of children are felt during and immediately following the act of abuse. The child endures pain and potential medical complications arising from physical harm, which, in severe cases, could even lead to death. The physical discomfort resulting from injuries like cuts, bruises, or burns, or from actions like whipping, kicking, punching, or strangulation, may eventually fade, yet the emotional trauma tends to persist long after the visible scars have healed.

The age at which the abuse takes place significantly influences the nature of the injuries and any lasting damage. Infants who are victims of physical abuse are at the highest risk of developing long-term physical complication, including neurological damage manifesting as tremors, lethargy, irritability, and vomiting. In more severe cases, physical abuse of children can result in seizures, permanent loss of sight or hearing, paralysis, mental and development delays, and, in extreme cases, death. The duration of the abuse also plays a crucial role with pronged abuse leading to more severe impacts on the child, irrespective of their age.

Moreover, the abuse can result in lifelong disabilities or brain injuries, cognitive delays, and profound emotional issues. Teens might resort to substance abuse, experience suicidal ideation, and demonstrate repetitive self-harming behaviours. They may struggle to form enduring friendships or relationships, haunted by the fear of repeated physical abuse.

Adult survivors of physical abuse in their childhood often bear the physical, emotional, and social repercussions of the abuse throughout their lives. Research indicates that such individuals are at an increased risk of developing mental illness, becoming homeless, engaging in criminal activities, and facing unemployment. These consequences pose a financial strain on communities and society at large, necessitating the allocation of resources towards social welfare programs funded through taxes and other revenue streams.

Family history of suicide

This refers to a situation where a family member has completed suicide, sometimes leaving with the reasons for their action unexplained to the family.

Having a family history of suicide has been identified as notably heightening the risk of suicide attempts across patients with a range of diagnoses, including schizophrenia, unipolar disorder, bipolar disorder, borderline personality disorder, depressive neurosis, and various other personality disorders.

How can this affect children/teens?

We examine the impact of losing a parent on children and teens.

When a child or teen loses a parent to suicide, it can act as a trigger for future suicide and psychiatric disorders. Developmental, environmental, and genetic factors most likely interact simultaneously to increase this risk.

Children and teens may have numerous queries regarding suicide, especially if someone in their family has taken their own life.

These questions might include:

- What is suicide?
- Did my action contribute to this event? Is it my fault?
- Could I have intervened to prevent the suicide?
- Should I have behaved differently?
- Will I also end my life through suicide?
- Are you going to commit suicide?

- If I commit suicide, will I reunite with my loved one?
- What should I tell my schoolmates?
- Why do I feel such profound sadness? Is this feeling everlasting?

After the death of a loved one, children may experience a range of emotions such as:

- Feeling abandoned
- Shock
- Sadness
- Anger
- Fear
- Guilt
- Confusion
- Depression
- Anxiety
- Feeling lost or empty

Children and teens often struggle with persistent intense grief. They tend to mourn in brief periods stretched over an extended timeframe. Their behaviour may switch between sorrow and normal play, causing confusion to both adults and themselves.

Unfortunately, due to the stigma and negative perceptions surrounding suicide, the grief experienced by survivors is often dismissed. This makes the grieving process even more challenging.

Here are some strategies to help children and teens navigate their grief:

- Ensure children and teens understand that their feelings are temporary and that they will not always feel this way. It's important to instil a sense of hope.

- Encourage children and teens to express their feelings. While some children and teens might be comfortable talking, others might prefer drawing or playing to explore their emotions. Listen attentively to what they say and observe what they leave unsaid.

- Acknowledge and validate children's and teen's emotions. Make supportive statements such as "I see that you're very sad" or "It's okay to feel angry."

Exposure to any sort of violence

Children can be exposed to many different types of violence as they grow up. Some examples are:

- Sexual abuse/assault
- Physical abuse/assault
- Domestic and family violence

- Neglect
- Schoolyard bullying

What is domestic and family violence?

Domestic violence has many aspects, including:

- Power and control are used to intentionally control or dominate their intimate partner/family member. The offender commonly uses threats, intimidation, and coercion to instil fear in their partner/victim.

- Physical abuse (as described above) can happen within a domestic relationship with parents, other family members, and intimate partners.

- Sexual abuse/assault (as described above) can also happen in the form of domestic violence amongst parents, other family members, and intimate partners.

- Emotional abuse can take place by using verbal abuse. Rejection occurs by constantly rejecting another's thoughts, ideas, and opinions. Gaslighting causes another person to doubt their own thoughts, feelings, and sanity by manipulating the truth and giving put-downs. Fear-building makes another person feel afraid, intimidated, or threatened. Emotional abuse can also take the form of isolation, financial abuse, bullying, and intimidation by purposely and repeatedly saying or doing things that are intended to hurt.

- Intimidation is used to frighten someone for fun or to act tough to get what they want.

- Social abuse can take the form of isolation from family, friends, work and/or getting family and friends to alienate the victim, trying to force the victim to move to an area with no support or family available, restricting the use of the car and/or phone, or stopping the victim from going out.

- Verbal abuse takes the form of coercion, threats, blame, name-calling, put-downs, swearing, humiliation, or screaming/shouting.

- Male privilege may be used to treat another person like a servant, make all the big decisions, act like the master of the castle, define men's and women's roles, destroy property or valued possessions, making threats regarding custody of their children, or making threats to kill oneself/the victim or another family member.

- Financial abuse takes the form of controlling or withholding money, preventing work or study, or theft.

- Stalking and/or harassment may be caused by following and watching the victim, phone and/or online harassment, GPS tracking to see where the victim is, being intimidating, or turning up at the victim's location or their house – particularly unexpectedly.

- Spiritual or religious abuse may take the form of stopping a person from practising their religious or spiritual beliefs, the perpetrator excusing their own violence and abuse, blaming the victim for the violence and abuse, or encouraging the victim to accept the violence and abuse.

- Psychological abuse creates fear by driving dangerously, possessing weapons, or giving angry looks.

- As you can see, many aspects of domestic violence can and do overlap. It's quite common to experience more than one type of violence at once.

What is neglect?

Some areas of neglect are:

- Not having physical needs met (shelter, food, clothing, hygiene, sleep)

- Not receiving affection from their main caregiver (cuddles, kisses, holding, tenderness, patience)

- Not feeling secure and safe (not being abandoned by parent/s, having consistent care, having appropriate boundaries, knowing who their actual parent/s are)

- Not having proper guidance while growing up (being taught life skills, values, and basic rights like having the right to say no, especially when feeling threatened or in an unsafe environment)

- Not being given an age-appropriate level of independence (being taught confidence, self-esteem, motivation, and safe methods of exploration when old enough to do things on their own)

- Not having the correct responsibilities given to them to help them learn (assigned appropriate chores, involved in age-appropriate decision-making)

- Not being shown the positive attitude that children need when growing up (encouragement, praise, and play)

- Not being accepted or receiving approval for their actions (understanding, appreciation, acceptance)

- Lack of education and support (having a consistent school setting and attendance, and encouragement, help, and support in learning)

What is schoolyard bullying?

Schoolyard bullying refers to the intentional psychological, emotional, or physical mistreatment of one student by another individual or a group. It takes place within the school premises or during the journey between school and home. This form of bullying encompasses actions such as peer group exclusion, intimidation, extortion, and acts of violence. It is important to note that not all children who experience schoolyard bullying will openly discuss it, particularly if they are the ones being targeted, as they fear the situation may escalate.

How do these types of violence affect children/teens?

Children and teens who experience violence often face various negative effects on their overall functioning, attitude, social competence, and school performance. They may have difficulties in basic coping and social skills, contributing to a decline in their self-esteem. The impact of violence is further intensified by factors like substance abuse mostly by teens, which exacerbates the negative outcomes. These individuals also have higher rates of anxiety, depression, other mental health problems, and even suicidal thoughts.

Bullying can significantly hinder academic progress as students who are targeted may develop a fear of standing out. Consequently, teachers may perceive them as low achievers or unmotivated learners, resulting in reduced attention and support. This perpetuates a cycle that further lowers their academic standing within the school.

Additionally, experiencing violence can contribute to the development of various issues, including depression, anxiety, sleep disturbances, challenges with forming healthy relationships, academic struggles, substance abuse, psychotic behaviour, antisocial behaviour, eating disorders, conduct disorders, and difficulties in obtaining and maintaining employment.

What is aggressive and disruptive behaviour?

Disruptive behaviour refers to any actions or conduct that creates difficulties for others. Aggressive behaviour, on the other hand, entails actions that have the potential to cause harm to someone else. Some instances of disruptive or aggressive behaviour include:

- Failing to adhere to school and household rules
- Exhibiting tantrums
- Demonstrating intense anger

How can this affect children/teens?

Aggressive and disruptive conduct can have a significant influence on a child's or teen's growth. Youngsters displaying signs of disruptive behaviour disorders may show a heightened tendency to enter into disputes, disobey requests, point fingers at others for their mistakes, purposefully bother others, or act out, diverging from the behaviour of their peers.

If these disruptive behaviours persist, the repercussions can be quite severe. These children may find themselves removed from the classroom, sent to the principal's office, or even suspended or expelled from school. As a result, these students miss out on valuable learning and social interaction opportunities.

Persistent aggression in the early years can lead to serious problems. It could be linked to mental disorders, poor social outcomes, and an accumulation of deficits, all of which could hinder the child's overall growth.

Moreover, aggressive and disruptive behaviour can jeopardize interpersonal relationships and increase the risk of physical harm from fights or risky behaviours like reckless driving.

The resulting strained relationships and physical injuries can have long-term detrimental effects.

Summary

The issue of suicide among young individuals is an alarming and serious one, securing its position as the second-most common cause of death in the age group of ten- to fourteen-year-olds. A vast majority of children and teens who attempt suicide are grappling with a significant mental health disorder, most frequently depression. This underscores the importance of vigilance in noticing any indications of suicidal thoughts or behaviours. The immediate response should involve seeking recognition, diagnosis, and treatment from mental health professionals who are trained at managing such scenarios.

While depression is often the mental health disorder most linked to suicidal ideation, it's important to realize that the picture can be more complex with other risk factors coming into play. The manner in which children and adolescents communicate their suicidal thoughts can also vary greatly. Some may be quite vocal about their feelings, others may remain silent, and some might only drop subtle hints. Therefore, parents need to be observant of warning signs. These can include seemingly innocuous behaviours such as gifting away cherished possessions or an abrupt loss of interest in future plans.

Establishing an open dialogue about suicide with children or adolescents is a daunting but crucial task. A trusting and safe environment should be fostered by parents to motivate their children to confide in them about their thoughts, and to facilitate the process of seeking professional help.

Safety should always be the top priority, and a mental health professional must be consulted without delay if there is any suspicion of suicidal ideation. In these trying circumstances, remaining calm is most important. Extreme emotional reactions could exacerbate the situation, creating more stress and fear for the child or teen.

Alongside suicidal tendencies, self-harm, also known as self-injury or self-mutilation, is another concerning behaviour. It entails intentionally inflicting harm upon oneself, not necessarily with a suicidal intention. It's essential to comprehend that self-harm doesn't automatically indicate a wish to end one's life. However, continuous self-injurious actions can heighten the risk of developing suicidal thoughts and behaviours in children and adolescents.

If parents or caregivers notice signs that their child is self-harming, immediate intervention is necessary. Instead of expressing condemnation, anger, sadness, guilt, or worry, support and assistance should be extended. The child or teen needs to feel safe and secure enough to confide their feelings and struggles to trustworthy individuals. The book aims to provide practical methods for parents and caregivers to help young individuals combat self-harm and suicidal ideation. If a parent or caregiver is having strong emotions around this, they too should seek help and assistance for themselves. However, as much as it is hard not to show these emotions in front of the child or teen, it is important to remove yourself from the situation by going to another room when you feel the need to express these emotions. Doing so in front of the child or teen could make them feel like they have done some wrong and may cause them to shut down even further than they have already.

Visible signs of self-harm to watch out for include observable cuts or scars, but these aren't the only indicators as children and teens may go to great lengths to conceal their injuries. Other forms of self-injury are also prevalent, such as head-banging, burning oneself, hair-pulling, or excessive scratching. The signs may not always be apparent, reinforcing the need for attentiveness and understanding.

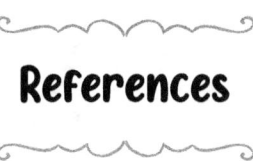

References

Colour Dream; Feeling Free: Survivors of Trauma

colourdreambooks.com

Centres for Disease Control and Prevention

cdc.gov/suicide/facts/index.html

Child and Adolescent Mental Health Services

camh.ca/en/health-info/guides-and-publications/when-a-parent-dies-by-suicide

www.ingramcontent.com/pod-product-compliance
Lightning Source LLC
LaVergne TN
LVHW021741060526
838200LV00052B/3393